Humphrey the Magic Frog to the Rescue

Volume 1

I0439741

Healthy Eating

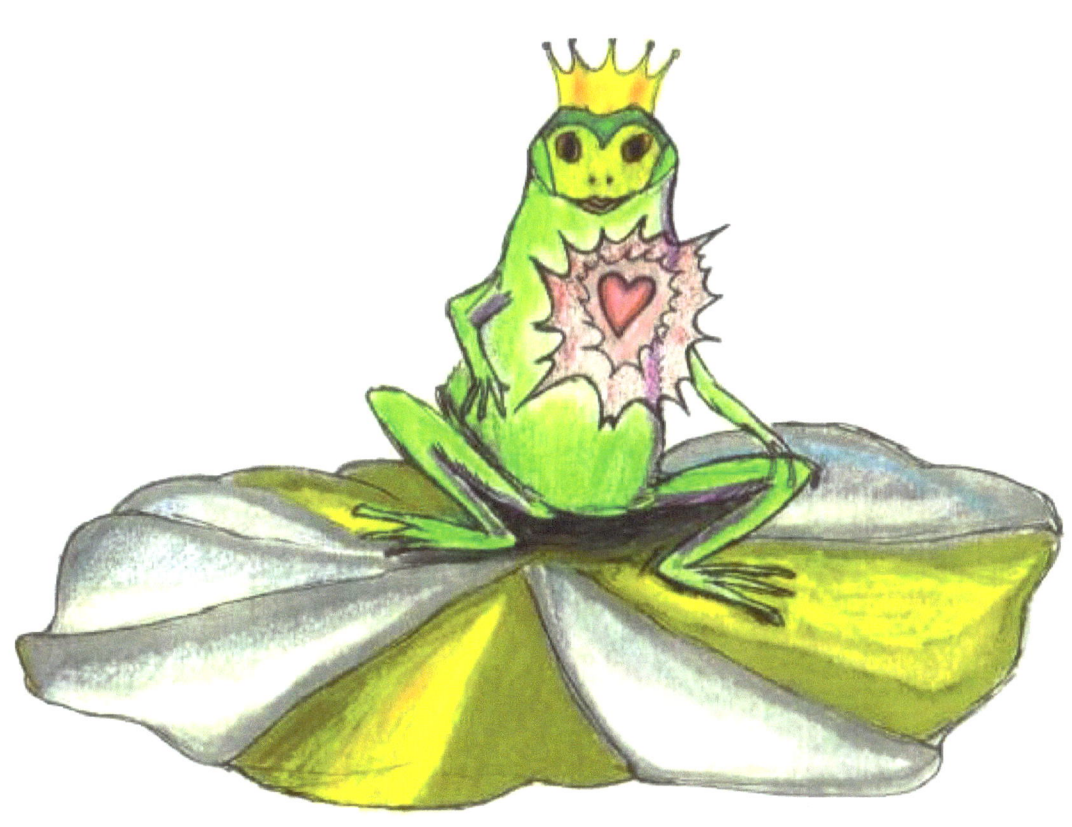

Table of Contents:

An Introduction to Humphrey the Magic Frog

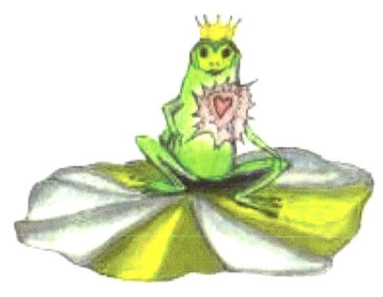

Humphrey the Magic Frog is a very unique and special frog. He is silvery-green and iridescent in color. Humphrey has a kind heart, a wonderful, all-knowing smile, a soft gentle voice, and a caring manner. His heart "glows" a bright shocking pink whenever he helps any animal-friend in need!

Humphrey lives in the wonderful world of Jasper Jungle on a silver and golden lily-pad in the center of Salem Pond. His silver and golden lily-pad gently glides to the surface of Salem Pond amid churning waters when called upon by any animal in need of his help.

All the animals, great and small, of land, sea, and air, know they can depend on Humphrey the Magic Frog to help them with their problems. All they need do is ask, and Humphrey appears at their side to help them. With their problems solved, Humphrey the Magic Frog smiles his all-knowing smile, taps his nose three times, taps his shocking pink heart three times, and vanishes from sight.

Through my series of stories, "Humphrey The Magic Frog to the Rescue," children ages Pre-K to Grade 4 will learn in a fun, entertaining way, simple solutions to the everyday problems they face using common sense, simple logic, and sometimes even "a wee bit of Humphrey magic!"

The 35 children's stories I have written with Humphrey the Magic Frog as my pivotal character are filled with important life-lessons for children. Some of the topics include: bullying, friendship, healthy eating, self-acceptance, adoption, family values, proper school behavior, and other life-lessons.

The stories are all filled with whimsical animal characters and every animal's friend, Humphrey the Magic Frog!

Humphrey and I hope you will invite us to put "a wee bit of Humphrey Magic" into your classrooms, libraries, and homes!

Peter Penguin's Portly Problem

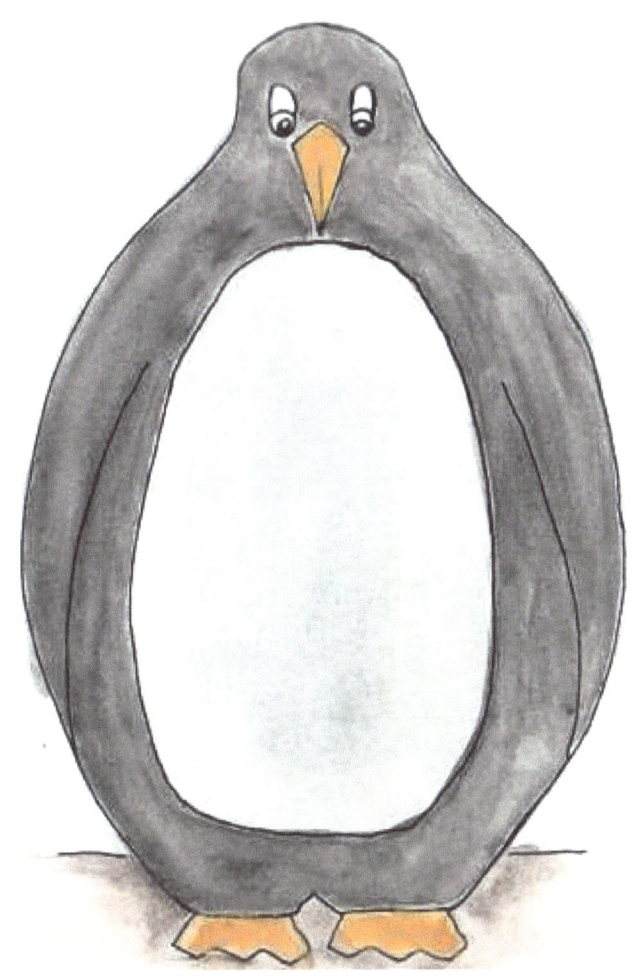

Picture by S. Kaz

Peter Penguin's Portly Problem

Peter Penguin Harrison was a very round, portly penguin. As long as he could remember, everyone had called him Portly Pete Penguin. Although Peter truly disliked being called Portly Pete Penguin, he'd simply smile and pretend to everyone that the name "Portly Pete" didn't bother him at all.

Yet, when called "Portly Pete" by anyone, Peter Penguin would go sadly into his bedroom and close the door. With his bedroom door closed, Peter Penguin would then begin munching and crunching all the cookies, candy, and junk-food his penguin hands could gather.

"MUNCH, MUNCH, CRUNCH, CRUNCH, GULP, GULP....

MUNCH, MUNCH, CRUNCH, CRUNCH, GULP, GULP."

Because of all his munching, crunching, and gulping on candy, cookies, and other snacks Peter Penguin Harrison became rounder and rounder with every passing day. One day, during his munching and crunching, Peter noticed his reflection in his bedroom mirror. Peter waddled up to the mirror and turned this way and that, that way and this. All of a sudden, he burst into tears.

"Oh my, look at me, look at me! What have I done? It is true! It is true! I am a round, round, portly, penguin! Oh, how will I ever fit into my new, birthday penguin suit in just five weeks?" cried a sad, sad Peter Penguin.

Peter turned from the bedroom mirror in horror and dashed to his bed, sliding beneath the covers to avoid the mirror's reflection. Peter remained beneath the covers crying silently until his tears ran out. As Peter cried and hid beneath the covers on his bed, he kept thinking and wishing, "Oh my, oh my, I wish someone could help me with my problem. I wish someone could help me."

Suddenly, Peter felt something touch his shoulder and someone gently call his name. "Peter, Peter what's wrong? It's Humphrey the Magic Frog. I arrived a few minutes ago to pay you a visit, but you were crying so loudly that you didn't hear me call your name. Please tell me what's wrong. You know I'll do all in my power to help you."

"Oh Humphrey, I am very afraid I am beyond all help. You see, in just five weeks I will be five years old, and I will be getting my very own first penguin suit. It is my one and only white penguin suit, and I must wear it for the rest of my life. And look at me, just look at me. No penguin suit in the world is going to fit me now. I am so round and portly. What can I do? Oh, what can I do?"

Humphrey the Magic Frog knowingly shook his head as he looked at Peter Penguin's bedroom floor. Humphrey saw that the entire bedroom floor was covered with empty candy wrappers, empty cookie boxes, empty potato chip and pretzel bags, and other empty packages of junk-food.

Humphrey noticed, too, that under Peter Penguin's bed, in his closet, under the bedroom rug, and even in every dresser drawer were more empty candy wrappers, boxes, and bags. Humphrey knew at once what must be done to help his sad friend, Peter Penguin.

"Ok, Peter," said Humphrey, "Dry your eyes and let's go for a walk to the park. I am sure we can come up with an answer to your problem."

And so, Peter and Humphrey walked and walked and walked. They walked for the longest time and neither said a word.

All of a sudden, Humphrey stopped. Humphrey then tapped his nose three times, tapped his heart three times, and shouted, "I've got it, Peter! I've got it! Just repeat these Eleven Magical Words of Wisdom after me. Come on, Peter, let me hear you sing!"

And Humphrey the Magic Frog began to sing:

♪ JIGGLE – JIGGLE – JOG ♪

♪ JIGGLE – JIGGLE – JOG ♪

♪ JIGGLE – JIGGLE ♪

♪ JIGGLE – JIGGLE – JOG! ♪

An excited Humphrey the Magic Frog called out to Peter Penguin, "Peter, the words are easy to remember, and don't just stand in one place as you sing the words -- **JOG**, **PETER, JOG**!"

"But," protested Peter, "how can singing a bunch of words help me fit into my penguin suit?"

"Listen, Peter. Three times a day for the next five weeks, you are to sing these Eleven Magical Words of Wisdom and jog around the house and town as you sing them.

And if you follow all my easy instructions, you have my promise that in just five weeks' time, on your very special birthday, you will fit perfectly into your new, beautiful penguin suit."

Humphrey the Magic Frog then told Peter Penguin that he must this very day stop secretly eating candy, chips, and other junk foods. Humphrey also told Peter that he must this very day begin eating only the healthy foods which his mother places on his plate at mealtimes.

Peter Penguin was then told by Humphrey the Magic Frog to eat lots of fresh vegetables such as peas, carrots, broccoli, cauliflower, spinach, potatoes, and lots of fresh fruits such as apples, oranges, peaches, pears, and grapes.

Humphrey the Magic Frog also told Peter Penguin to eat fish, cheese, beans, eggs, and grains like bread and cereal, and to drink milk, juice, and water each and every day.

Most important of all, Peter Penguin was told by Humphrey the Magic Frog to stop secretly eating cookies, candy, chips, and other junk-foods.

After telling Peter Penguin these very important rules for becoming a healthy, happy penguin, Humphrey the Magic Frog's heart began to glow and glow a shocking-pink color.

Humphrey the Magic Frog then smiled his all-knowing smile, tapped his nose three times, tapped his shocking-pink heart three times, and *VANISHED* from sight!

Peter Penguin was confused. He searched everywhere for his friend, Humphrey the Magic Frog, but he could not find him. Humphrey had simply vanished! Peter shook his head. He then remembered all of Humphrey's advice and all that Humphrey had told him he must do. "It's worth a try," thought Peter Penguin. So, every single day for five weeks, Peter Penguin followed all of Humphrey the Magic Frog's instructions.

Three times every day Peter Penguin jogged about the house and town singing Humphrey the Magic Frog's Eleven Magical Words of Wisdom:

♪ JIGGLE – JIGGLE – JOG ♪

♪ JIGGLE – JIGGLE – JOG ♪

♪ JIGGLE – JIGGLE ♪

♪ JIGGLE – JIGGLE – JOG! ♪

Every single day as instructed by Humphrey the Magic Frog, Peter Penguin could be found singing and jogging, singing and jogging. He jogged around the house, down the street, up the block, and all through town.

Peter Penguin also remembered Humphrey the Magic Frog's Words of Wisdom and began eating healthy, delicious foods such as fruits, vegetables, fish, grains, milk, water, and juice each day, and Peter even stopped secretly eating junk-foods in his bedroom.

And five weeks later on Peter Penguin's fifth birthday, Peter Penguin Harrison was wearing his beautiful, sleek, new white penguin suit. Humphrey the Magic Frog had truly kept his promise! Portly Peter Penguin was now a healthy, sleek, happy penguin.

Peter Penguin is no longer called Portly Pete by anyone. And when one of his penguin friends called him "Sir Peter Penguin Harrison" because he looked so stylish, sleek, and healthy, Peter Penguin simply shook his head, smiled, and said, "Just call me Pete."

Humphrey the Magic Frog taught Peter Penguin **two very important lessons** which changed his life....

Peter Penguin learned the **importance of eating healthy foods** such as fruits, vegetables, beans, fish, grains like bread and cereal, cheese, juice, milk, and water.

Peter Penguin also learned the **importance of exercise** and happily sings Humphrey's Eleven Magical Words of Wisdom each and every time he walks, strolls, or jogs about the neighborhood:

♪ JIGGLE – JIGGLE – JOG ♪

♪ JIGGLE – JIGGLE – JOG ♪

♪ JIGGLE – JIGGLE ♪

♪ JIGGLE – JIGGLE – JOG! ♪

Always remember the words of a Magic Frog named Humphrey:

RIBBIT, RIBBIT…EAT HEALTHY FOODS!

RIBBIT…DON'T JUST SIT THERE!

MOVE! SING! DANCE! JOG!

Henry Hippo's Frail Tale

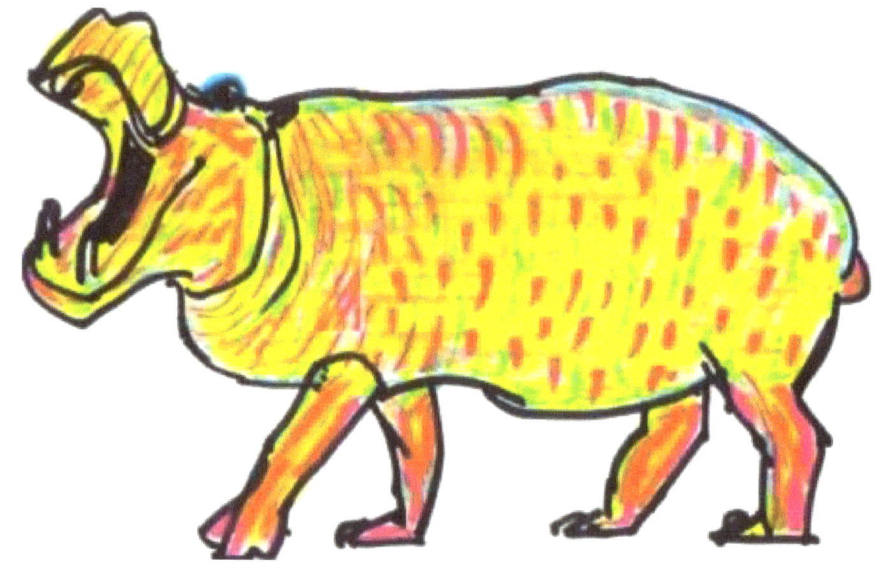

Picture by D. Jackovino

Henry Hippo's Frail Tale

"That's the house of stay-at-home, hide-in-the-house, no-friends-at-all Henry Hippo," laughed all the neighborhood hippos whenever they walked by Henry Hippo's house.

When Henry Hippo heard all the hippo laughter, he would close all the windows, pull down the shades, and hide in the darkness. Truly, Henry Hippo was a thin, frail, so very weak-in-the-knees, sad little hippo.

And even though he liked to eat, (and he sure did eat!) poor, thin, frail, so very weak-in-knees Henry Hippo could not gain one ounce of healthy-hippo weight. All the other hippos in Hippo Land laughed and laughed at poor Henry Hippo for he was so very thin, so very frail, and so very weak-in-the-knees.

Day after day, week after week, Henry Hippo tried and tried to gain healthy-hippo weight. However, poor, thin, frail, so very weak-in-the-knees Henry Hippo got only thinner and thinner and weaker and weaker.

Henry Hippo drank soda pop and ate marshmallows all day and all night long to try to gain weight, but he didn't gain any healthy hippo weight. Henry Hippo was so very sad. He cried and cried. He tried and tried. However, sadly to say, poor, thin, frail, very weak in the knees Henry Hippo simply could not gain one ounce of healthy-hippo weight.

Henry Hippo was so very thin and frail that he even had trouble standing. He was so very thin and frail that he even had a hard time holding up his sad-eyed, heavy hippo head.

Poor, sad, thin, frail, weak-in-the-knees Henry Hippo even had a hard time sitting. But, worst of all, poor, thin, frail, very weak-in-the-knees Henry Hippo had a hard time sleeping. Henry Hippo stayed up night after sleepless night. For you see, Henry Hippo's empty stomach was so very, very noisy that he could not get any sleep. All night long, hour after hour, Henry Hippo's empty stomach would **growl, hiss, and gurgle, growl, hiss, and gurgle.** And all the noise from his empty stomach kept poor Henry Hippo awake, night after sleepless night.

Henry Hippo knew he needed help. But poor, thin, frail, weak-in-the- knees Henry Hippo was too sleepy and too weak to visit the local animal doctor for help.

One sunny day, Henry Hippo was visited by his friend, Samuel Snake. When Samuel saw poor, frail, weak-in-the-knees Henry Hippo, he knew at once that Henry Hippo needed help. Deeply concerned, Samuel Snake slithered seven miles to Salem Pond and searched for Humphrey the Magic Frog. Samuel Snake knew that Humphrey the Magic Frog always helped animals in need, and Henry Hippo truly was an animal who needed help with his problem.

When Samuel Snake arrived at the edge of Salem Pond, he quietly called out three times:

Hummm-Hummm-Free!

Hummm-Hummm-Free!

Hummm-Hummm-Free!

As Samuel Snaked chanted these words, the waters of Salem Pond began to churn and churn. From the center of the churning waters a beautiful silver and gold lily pad arose to the surface of the water. Sitting atop the beautiful silver and gold lily pad was Humphrey the Magic Frog. In a flash, Humphrey the Magic Frog was sitting next to Samuel Snake at the edge of Salem Pond.

"Yes, my friend, Samuel Snake. I heard you calling out to me. How may I help you?" Samuel Snake then told Humphrey the Magic Frog all about his poor, sad, frail, weak-in-the-knees friend Henry Hippo, and begged for his help. When Samuel Snake finished telling Humphrey his sad story about Henry Hippo, Samuel Snake was crying. Samuel Snake shook and cried, shook and cried.

"Stop crying, friend Samuel Snake. I promise you I will help your poor, frail, weak-in-the-knees friend, Henry Hippo. Never fear! Humphrey the Magic Frog is here!" And with those words, Humphrey the Magic Frog tapped his nose three times, tapped his heart, and vanished from sight.

Within several magical seconds, Humphrey the Magic Frog was sitting at the foot of Henry Hippo's bed. With one quick look at poor, frail, weak-in-the-knees Henry Hippo sitting on his bed, Humphrey knew that Henry Hippo truly needed his help.

"Hello, Henry," said Humphrey the Magic Frog in a gentle voice. "Your friend Samuel Snake is very worried about you. He came to Salem Pond and told me of your problem. After hearing his story, I promised him that I would help you."

"Oh my, oh my, I'm so glad you have come to help me, Humphrey. I really do need help. Please help me, Oh, please help me," cried Henry Hippo.

"Rest for a few minutes," said Humphrey in a gentle and caring voice. "I will be right back." Humphrey then got up from Henry Hippo's bed and began to walk from room to room to room. Humphrey looked into all the cupboards and saw that they were all filled to the brim with soda pop and marshmallows. He looked into the refrigerator and saw that it, too, was filled to the brim with soda pop and marshmallows. Humphrey also looked into all of the closets of the entire house and saw that they were also filled to the brim with soda pop and marshmallows.

"Why, my goodness," Humphrey the Magic Frog exclaimed, as he discovered that even Henry Hippo's bathtub and kitchen sink were filled to the brim with cans and bottles of soda pop and marshmallows of every size and color. "I see, I see," exclaimed Humphrey the Magic Frog, as he returned to Henry Hippo's bedroom.

When Humphrey the Magic Frog reached Henry Hippo's bedroom, he knew what must be done. Humphrey the Magic Frog tapped his nose three times, tapped his heart, and smiled his famous, big, knowing, wonderful, magical smile. As Humphrey tapped his heart, it began to glow and glow a bright shocking pink color.

In a very caring voice, Humphrey quietly said to Henry Hippo, "Henry Hippo, you must listen to my words, and do as I instruct you to do. If you do everything I instruct you to do, I promise, you will soon become a strong, healthy, happy hippo." Humphrey the Magic Frog then touched Henry Hippo's shoulder and quietly said these **Thirteen Words of Wisdom** to his friend, as his shocking pink heart began to glow:

"MY FRIEND HENRY, YOU SHOULD KNOW.....

EATING HEALTHY FOODS.....

WILL HELP YOU GROW!"

As Humphrey repeated his **Thirteen Words of Wisdom**, Henry Hippo sadly looked at Humphrey the Magic Frog and said, "Humphrey, How can a bunch of words help me? I eat so much now. Yet, I am still a thin, frail, weak-in-the-knees hippo."

Humphrey looked kindly into Henry Hippo's sad, confused, frightened eyes. Humphrey smiled his warm, knowing smile and said, "Friend Henry Hippo, you must, this very day, this very second, stop eating only soda pop and marshmallows. You must, this very day, eat a well-balanced and healthy diet."

Then Humphrey the Magic Frog continued, "Henry, you must begin eating vegetables such as beans, broccoli, carrots, and cauliflower. You must also eat fruits such as pears, apples, oranges, grapes and bananas, and healthy grains such as bread and cereal. And don't forget to drink milk, juice, and water, too. If you follow my advice, you will become a strong, healthy, happy hippo in a very short time."

After speaking those final words to Henry Hippo, Humphrey the Magic Frog's heart turned a shocking-pink color as he tapped his nose three times, tapped his shocking pink heart and *VANISHED* from sight!

Henry Hippo slowly sat up in his bed. He looked around, but Humphrey was gone. Henry then remembered Humphrey's words of advice, and he knew what he must do.

Henry Hippo slowly got out of bed and walked from room to room collecting all the soda pop cans and bottles in his house. He then put them all into large plastic garbage bags. Next, he collected all the bags and boxes of marshmallows from every room in his house and put them all into large plastic garbage bags as well.

Henry Hippo then took a deep breath and slowly, ever so slowly, pulled and pulled all the large, plastic garbage bags to the front of his house to be picked up by the garbage patrol the very next day.

On that very same day, Henry Hippo began to eat a healthy, well-balanced diet. He ate a healthy breakfast, a healthy lunch, and a healthy dinner each and every day. Henry Hippo also ate healthy snacks of fresh fruits and vegetables each day.

And as promised by his friend, Humphrey the Magic Frog, in a very short time Henry Hippo was transformed into a healthy, happy, hippo.

Henry Hippo now leaves his house each day and romps and plays with Samuel Snake and his many hippo friends!

And Henry Hippo has never forgotten his friend, Humphrey the Magic Frog, or Humphrey's Thirteen Words of Wisdom:

MY FRIEND HENRY, YOU SHOULD KNOW.....

EATING HEALTHY FOODS.....

WILL HELP YOU GROW!

Matthew Mouse:

The Case of the Shrinking Clothes

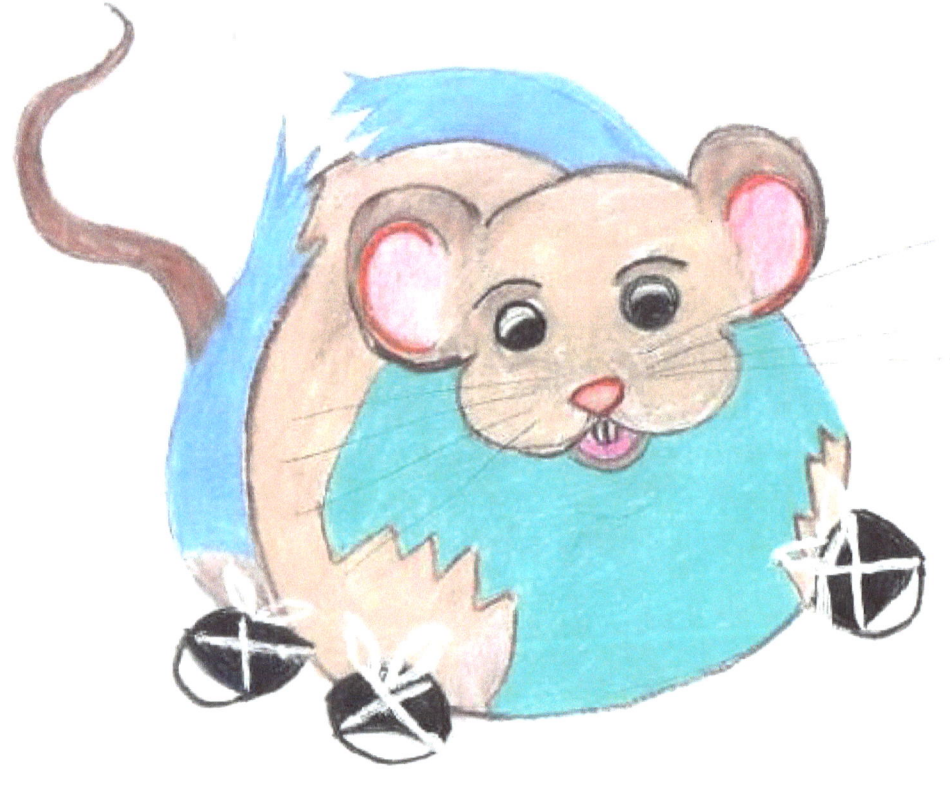

Picture by Hannah Fanelli

Matthew Mouse:

The Case of the Shrinking Clothes

Matthew Mouse was a very kind, friendly mouse. He was also a very popular mouse. Whenever there was a mouse-party in Mouseville, Matthew Mouse would always be invited.

"Hey, Matt, come to my house, tonight. We're having a mouse-get-together. I hope to see you, then," said Tom Mouse, one of Matt's many close mouse-friends.

"I'll be serving cheese, cheese, cheese," laughed Tom Mouse, "and everyone knows what a cheese-lover you are, Matt," Tom said, as he hung up the phone.

"A mouse-get-together at Tom's," smiled Matthew Mouse. "Now, what can I wear?" he thought as he searched his closet for the perfect outfit.

"Hmmmm, my black pants and black and white shirt would be the perfect clothes to wear," thought a smiling Matthew Mouse.

"Yes," Matthew Mouse continued, "I'll wear these clothes to the party at Tom's tonight," said Matthew Mouse, as he ever so carefully placed the pants and shirt on a nearby chair.

Matthew Mouse was indeed a very popular mouse with many good friends and lots and lots of wonderful clothes. But, our friend, Matthew Mouse, had one bad habit. He would only eat **CHEESE** and nothing else.

Matthew Mouse would eat cheese for breakfast, cheese for lunch, cheese for dinner and snacks, and nothing else. Matthew Mouse would eat cream cheese from a giant spoon and nothing else.

Matthew Mouse would eat large chunks of Swiss, mozzarella, and cheddar cheese and nothing else. Matthew Mouse would eat slices of American cheese and parmesan cheese by the pound and nothing else.

Matthew Mouse truly was a super-duper-lover-of-cheese!

He never ate any fruit. "No, thank you; no apples, peaches, plums, grapes, melon, or any other fruit for me. Just give me a slice of cheese, please," Matthew Mouse would say with a wide smile.

He never ate any vegetables. "No thank you; no broccoli, spinach, beets, tomatoes, olives, lettuce, beans, or any other vegetable for me. Just give me a chunk of cheese, please," Matthew Mouse would say with a wide smile.

He never ate grains, chicken, turkey, or any type of fish. Matthew only ate cheese.

As for dairy products, Matthew Mouse would only eat **CHEESE**.

Why, Matthew Mouse loved cheese so-much that he even wrote a poem about it...

MOUSE MATT'S ODE TO CHEESE

I'M A MOUSE, AS YOU CAN SEE.

I LOVE CHEESE AND CHEESE LOVES ME.

CHEESE IS THE ONLY FOOD FOR ME.

YES, CHEESE IS THE ONLY FOOD FOR ME!

Later that day, when Matthew Mouse tried to put on his black pants and black and white shirt to go to the party, they did not fit. They were both too small to wear. **"My goodness!"** said Matthew Mouse in a surprised voice. **"My clothes have SHRUNK!"** he said in disbelief.

"I guess I'll just have to wear something else to the party," Matthew Mouse said with a sigh. Matthew Mouse then scooted about the house looking for the perfect clothes to wear to Mouse Tom's party that night.

First, Matthew Mouse tried on his collection of pants. He first tried on his green pants. **"Rip, Rip, Rip"** went his green pants as he tried to pull them over his legs.

Then Matthew reached for his red pants. Again, **"Rip, Rip, Rip"** went his red pants.

The very same thing happened with his navy pants, his orange pants, his purple pants, his gray pants, his white pants, and his favorite pair of yellow pants. **"Rip, Rip, Rip"** was the sound that echoed in his ears!

"Oh, no, all of my beautiful pants have **SHRUNK!"** Matthew Mouse called out in horror.

Matthew then ran to his prized shirt collection in his closet and began to try on all his shirts. He first tried on his white shirt. **"Pop, Pop, Pop"** went all the buttons on his white shirt!

He then tried on his three blue shirts and, again, **"Pop, Pop, Pop"** went all the buttons on all his blue shirts!

The very same thing happened when he tried on his green shirts, his orange shirts, his black shirts, his red shirts, and his very favorite olive colored shirt, which had always been a bit too large to wear. The sound he heard over and over was **"Pop, Pop, Pop"** as the buttons flew from his shirts and fell to the floor!

"No! No! No! No!" screamed Matthew Mouse in his loudest, largest mouse-voice, "My shirts, my beautiful shirts have all **SHRUNK**, too! What am I to do? I've nothing at all to wear. How did this terrible thing happen?"

"Oh, my cheese-goodness, what am I to do, now?" asked a sad, sad Matthew Mouse. "I wish there were someone out there who could help me," Matt Mouse said in a sad, tired voice. He sadly walked to his bed, wrapped himself in his large yellow and green bed sheets, and said, "Well, at least there is something that still fits me. My bed sheets haven't **"SHRUNK**," he said with sad and tear-filled eyes. He then hid his head under his sheets, closed his tear-filled eyes, and fell asleep.

A short time later, as Matthew Mouse slept, he heard his name being called out in a kind and gentle voice. "Matthew Mouse, Matthew Mouse, wake up, my friend. I am Humphrey the Magic Frog. I heard your wish, and I have come to help you with your problem," said the caring voice.

"Problem? What Problem?" asked a sleepy Matthew Mouse in his bravest voice as he rubbed his tear-stained eyes. "Give me a chunk of cheese," said Matthew Mouse. "Problems. I have no problems at all."

Humphrey the Magic Frog smiled his all-knowing smile, looked around the room, and said in a kindly voice, "Matthew, it looks to me as if you've had some sort of rain-shower of clothes."

"Oh, that," said Matthew Mouse with a deep sigh, "They're just my shrunken clothes."

"Hmmmm, so all of your clothes have shrunk and no longer fit you," said Humphrey the Magic Frog. That's easy to fix," continued Humphrey Frog.

"Easy to fix, you say, Mr. Frog. How?" asked a rather sleepy and confused Matt Mouse as he rubbed his tired eyes.

"Well, since all of your clothes have shrunk, all we have to do is shrink you. That way, all your clothes will fit you again," said Humphrey smiling his famous all-knowing smile.

"What!? What do you mean? How can you possibly shrink me? I'm not a piece of clothing. I'm a real, live mouse. I'm made of flesh and bones, and I even have mouse-whiskers. How can you shrink me?" asked a very confused Matthew Mouse.

"Well," said Humphrey the Magic Frog, "You can begin to shrink yourself in a very simple, healthy way by eating the proper foods each day. **You can still eat some cheese, but you must also eat other healthy foods, as well," said Humphrey.**

Humphrey continued, "Instead of eating four slices of Swiss cheese, eat one slice of cheese and some broccoli."

"Instead of eating twelve spoonfuls of parmesan cheese, eat a sprinkle of parmesan cheese and a piece of chicken, turkey, fish, or an egg. Instead of eating a large chunk of cheddar cheese, eat a small slice of cheddar cheese with an apple or peach," said a smiling Humphrey the Magic Frog.

Humphrey continued in his matter-of-fact voice, "Matthew, you must stop eating only cheese all the time. You must begin eating fruits such as apples, pears, peaches, grapes, and melons. You must also begin eating vegetables such as broccoli, spinach, lettuce, beets, squash, and carrots just to name a few. And in no time at all, I promise you, that you will be wearing all your wonderful clothes on your wonderful, strong, healthy body," said Humphrey Frog.

"But, "I'm a mouse and I love **CHEESE**," Matthew Mouse said in his most serious voice.

Humphrey the Magic Frog said in a matter-of-fact voice, "Matthew, you can still have some cheese in your diet, but having only cheese for every meal, every single day is not a healthy idea."

Humphrey then smiled his all-knowing smile and said, "Matthew, I know how you love to sing. Please, sing these **Twenty-One Words of Wisdom with me**."

♪ SHRINKING IN SIZE ♪

♪ WILL BE EASY... YOU WILL SEE ♪

♪ IF YOU EAT THE PROPER FOODS ♪

♪ HEALTHY AND TRIM YOU WILL BE ♪

When they had finished singing, Humphrey the Magic Frog smiled and said to Matthew Mouse, "Matthew, sing these Twenty-One Words of Wisdom; eat healthy foods such as vegetables, fruits, grains, fish, poultry, and dairy; eat less cheese each day; and before you know it, you will fit into all of your wonderful clothes and become a happy, healthy, party-going mouse once more."

With those final words spoken, Humphrey the Magic Frog smiled his famous all-knowing smile, tapped his nose three times, tapped his heart which now glowed a bright shocking-pink three times, and *VANISHED*!

"Wow, A vanishing frog! If a frog is magic enough to vanish, I'd sure better listen to him," smiled Matthew Mouse.

That very same day, Matthew Mouse began taking Humphrey the Magic Frog's advice. He began eating healthy vegetables such as spinach, broccoli, squash, peas, carrots, lettuce, and many other vegetables.

He began eating healthy fruits such as bananas, peaches, plums, apples, grapes, melons, and many other fruits.

Matthew Mouse also began eating healthy grains such as whole wheat pasta, cereals, and whole wheat bread. He began eating healthy dairy products such as cottage cheese, yogurt, and milk. Matthew also ate just a tiny bit of cheese from time to time.

Matthew Mouse also ate chicken, turkey, and fish at least twice a week.

As promised by Humphrey the Magic Frog, in a very short time, Matthew Mouse was once again wearing his wonderful collection of once shrunken clothing.

Matthew Mouse is now a healthy, happy, handsome, well-dressed mouse, and every single day you can hear him singing in his happiest-mouse voice:

♪ SHRINKING IN SIZE ♪

♪ WILL BE EASY… YOU WILL SEE ♪

♪ IF YOU EAT THE PROPER FOODS ♪

♪ HEALTHY AND TRIM YOU WILL BE ♪

♪ THANK YOU, THANK YOU, MY FRIEND HUMPHREY ♪

Caldora Cat:

The Kitten Who Refused to Drink Milk

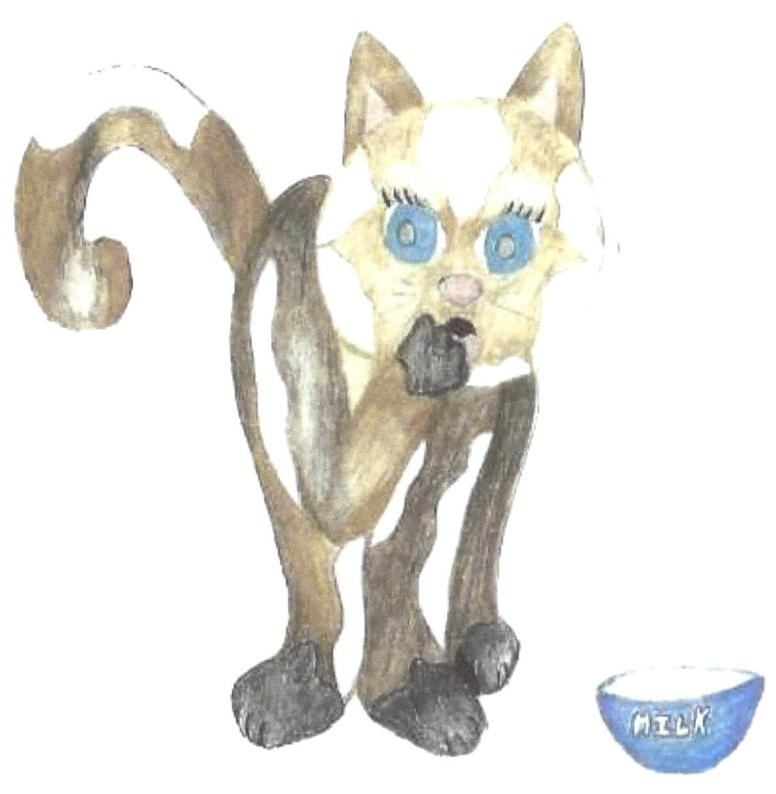

Picture by Hannah Fanelli

Caldora Cat:
The Kitten Who Refused to Drink Milk

Everyone knows how important it is to drink milk. Milk has calcium and calcium helps us grow strong bones and strong teeth. Calcium also helps us move our muscles and bend, skip, stretch, jump, climb, run, and dance.

Young cats and kittens of every shape, size, and color love to drink milk. Young cats and kittens love to drink warm milk and cold milk. Young cats and kittens love to drink whole milk, 2% milk, 1% milk, and skim-milk. Young cats and kittens drink milk out of tiny dishes, tiny plates, and tiny bowls with their names printed on them.

"SIP, SIP, SIP.   SIP, SIP, SIP.   SIP. SIP, SIP."

Most young cats and kittens truly love milk.

But then, there is Caldora Kitten...

Caldora Kitten is a beautiful brown and white kitten with black paws, a brown and white tail, and beautiful blue eyes. Caldora Kitten is kind and considerate to all her friends and loves her mom very much. Caldora Kitten always obeys her mom. Yet, there is one very important thing which Caldora Kitten always refuses to do for her mom.

Caldora Kitten refuses to drink milk or eat dairy products of any kind. And no matter how hard Rosa Cat tries to get her daughter Caldora to drink milk, Caldora always shakes her head, puts her left paw over her mouth, and says, "No! No! Not me! No milk or dairy products for me, Mom!"

Rosa Cat loves her daughter-kitten very much and wants her to grow-up to be a strong and healthy cat. She worries about Caldora not drinking milk or eating any dairy products. Caldora Kitten is not allergic to milk or dairy products; yet, she simply refuses to drink milk or eat dairy products at any of her meals.

"Mom, I'm fine. I Can Stretch! I Can Crawl! I Can Run! I Can Leap! I Can Climb the tallest trees! And I Can Dance! I don't need to drink any silly old milk, or eat any silly old dairy products. I don't need all that Calcium stuff. You worry too much," smiles Caldor Kitten.

That night before going to sleep, Rosa Cat looked out the window in her bedroom and said in a quiet voice, "I so wish someone could help me with Caldora. I wish someone could help me with my problem." Rosa then turned from the window and went to bed.

The very next morning, Rosa Cat heard someone knocking on her front door.

**KNOCK. KNOCK. KNOCK.
KNOCK. KNOCK. KNOCK***

Rosa walked to the front door and called out, "Yes? Who is it?"

A quiet, gentle voice said through the locked door, "I am Humphrey the Magic Frog, Rosa, and I have come to help you with your daughter Caldora." When Rosa Cat opened the door, she was greeted by a smiling, iridescent silver and green frog.

"Hello, Rosa, I heard your wish last night for help with your kitten-daughter, Caldora. I know that she refuses to drink milk or eat any dairy products, and I have come to teach her how important it is for a growing kitten to have Calcium in her diet," smiled Humphrey the Magic Frog.

Humphrey the Magic Frog then smiled his all-knowing smile and said to Rosa Cat, "I promise you, Rosa, that I will have Caldora drinking milk and eating dairy products this very day."

"Oh, Humphrey, I do hope so. Please come in and sit with me, and we can both enjoy a bowl of berries and cream while we wait for Caldora to come home.

Humphrey the Magic Frog smiled at Rosa Cat and said, "Why thank you, Rosa. I love berries and cream." Humphrey the Magic Frog then followed Rosa Cat into her kitchen, and together they enjoyed a large helping of berries and cream at Rosa's kitchen table.

As Rosa Cat and Humphrey the Magic Frog finished their last spoonful of berries and cream, the front door opened and Caldora Kitten walked into the room. "Hi, Mom, I see you have company," smiled Caldora.

"Hello, dear. This is my friend, Humphrey Frog," said a smiling Rosa Cat.

"Hello, Mr. Frog, it's nice to meet you," smiled Caldora.

"Hello, Caldora, it's so very nice to meet you, too. I just learned from your mom that you are a kitten who doesn't like to drink milk or eat any dairy products," said a smiling Humphrey the Magic Frog.

"Yep, that's me. I don't ever drink any milk. And I don't ever eat any dairy products," said a smiling Caldora Kitten.

Humphrey the Magic Frog shook his head, looked at Caldora Kitten and Rosa Cat, and said, "Hmmmm, I see. Caldora, my legs are a bit stiff from sitting too long, and I really need to take a long walk. Would you walk with me to the local park?" asked Humphrey Frog as he rubbed his left knee.

Caldora Kitten smiled and said, "Sure, Mr. Frog. I love the park. I walk there all the time."

Caldora Kitten and Humphrey the Magic Frog then both smiled at Rosa Cat and left the house for their walk. But before leaving the house, Caldora gave her mom a big hug and said, "Be right back mom. I am going for a walk to the park with your friend, Mr. Frog."

Rosa Cat smiled at her daughter Caldora and looking at Humphrey the Magic Frog said, "Have a good time and enjoy your walk together."

As they walked to the park, Humphrey asked, "Caldora, can we take longer steps as we walk? It will really help my stiff leg."

"Sure. I can do that," smiled Caldora. So, Caldora Kitten began to take long kitten-steps as she walked. And Humphrey the Magic Frog began to take long frog-steps as he walked.

All of a sudden, Caldora Kitten called out in a loud voice, "Stop! Stop, Mr. Frog! It hurts! It hurts when I take long kitten-steps. What's wrong with me?"

"Hmmmmm, I'm not quite sure. Why don't we take shorter steps as we walk to the park and see if that helps," said Humphrey. So Humphrey the Magic Frog and Caldora Kitten took short steps and continued to walk to the park.

Humphrey then saw a tall maple tree. "Caldora, can you climb to the top branch of that maple tree?" Humphrey asked.

"Sure, I can do that. I climb trees all the time. I'm a great tree-climber," smiled Caldora Kitten.

Caldora walked to the maple tree and started to climb to the very top branch. Caldora climbed to the first branch of the maple tree. Caldora climbed to the second branch of the maple tree. But when Caldora reached for the third branch of the maple tree, she called out in a loud voice, "Ouch! It Hurts! It Hurts! What's wrong with me?" Caldora Kitten then slowly climbed down from the tree and sadly walked away.

Humphrey the Magic Frog then said in a quiet, concerned voice, "Caldora, let's sit together on the grass and rest for a few minutes."

After resting on the grass for a few minutes, Humphrey said, "Caldora, we can walk to the park or we can walk back to your home. What would you like to do?"

"I want to walk to the park, Mr. Frog. I'm just fine," said Caldora Kitten. So Humphrey and Caldora Kitten got up from the grass, dusted themselves off, and continued their walk to the park.

When they reached the park, Caldora Kitten saw Ms. Lu's Dance Group. All the kittens in the dance group were dancing, smiling, and having fun.

Caldora Kitten smiled brightly and said, "I can dance like that, Mr. Frog. Watch me dance!" Caldora Kitten then ran across the grass and began to dance with the other kitten dancers. Ms. Lu watched Caldora as she danced with her kitten dance group. Ms. Lu smiled and said, "Hello, Caldora. It's so nice to see you. You are a very good dancer. Have fun!"

Ms. Lu then turned to her class and said, "Class, it's time for us to dance, dance, dance! Let's begin our warm-up exercises:

REACH AND STRETCH!   REACH AND STRETCH!

BEND!   BEND!   BEND!   BEND!

DIP!   DIP!   DIP!   DIP!

BOW!   BOW!   BOW!   BOW!"

"This is such fun," said Caldora Kitten as she danced with Ms. Lu's Dance Group.

A smiling Caldora Kitten danced with the other dancing kittens for several seconds when all of a sudden.....

CALDORA KITTEN STOPPED DANCING!

SHE STOPPED BENDING!

SHE STOPPED DIPPING!

SHE STOPPED REACHING!

SHE STOPPED STRETCHING!

SHE STOPPED BOWING!

CALDORA KITTEN SIMPLY STOPPED!!!

A sad Caldora Kitten walked away from the dance group with her head down. She walked over to where Humphrey Frog was sitting on the grass.

Humphrey said in a soft voice, "Why have you stopped dancing, Caldora? You looked so very happy as you danced."

"What am I to do, Mr. Frog? I can't climb trees. I can't take long steps when I walk. I can't bend and stretch when I dance. What's wrong with me?" cried Caldora Kitten as she threw herself down on the grass and cried her biggest, saddest, kitten-tears. Caldora Kitten cried and cried and cried.

"Caldora, please stop crying. It makes me so sad to see you cry. I can help you if you will let me," said Humphrey the Magic Frog.

"I will do anything you say, Mr. Frog. Please tell me what I must do," cried Caldora Kitten.

"Caldora, the answer is very simple. It is a word you know very well, but don't like very much. The word is **MILK**," said Humphrey the Magic Frog.

"Milk! Yick! No! No! No!" shouted Caldora Kitten in her loudest kitten-voice.

"Caldora, to be strong and healthy you must begin to drink milk each day. Milk contains CALCIUM and you need CALCIUM in your daily diet in order to have strong bones and strong teeth. CALCIUM also helps you move, stretch, bend, climb, and dance," said Humphrey Frog.

"Where can I get this important CALCIUM stuff?" asked Caldora.

Humphrey the Magic Frog smiled at Caldora Kitten and said, "Caldora, you can get CALCIUM in many, many ways. You can get Calcium by eating dairy products such as hard cheese, cottage cheese, buttermilk, yogurt, and ice cream. You can get CALCIUM by eating green leafy vegetables such as broccoli, spinach, kale, and lettuce. You can also get CALCIUM by eating salmon and sardines," said Humphrey Frog.

"No! No! You said I had to drink milk and I simply can't drink milk," cried Caldora Kitten.

"Caldora, let's try something," said Humphrey the Magic Frog. "Please close you eyes and repeat after me:

"MILK IS PURRRR-FECT!

MILK IS PURRRR-FECT!

MILK IS PURRRR-FECT!"

Caldora Kitten closed her eyes and said,

"MILK IS PURRRR-FECT.

MILK IS PURRRR-FECT.

MILK IS PURRRR-FECT."

Humphrey smiled at Caldora Kitten and said, "Caldora, you don't have to change the foods you eat in long, long kitten-steps. You can change the foods you eat in tiny, tiny kitten-steps. You start by drinking just a few drops of milk and eating just one tiny spoonful of yogurt the first day. Then slowly, ever so slowly, you add a tiny bit more each day," smiled Humphrey.

"Sure. I can do that, Mr. Frog. I promise to start drinking milk this very night at dinner. I also promise to eat a tiny bit of yogurt, too," said a smiling Caldora Kitten.

Caldora Kitten then smiled her biggest, brightest kitten-smile and said, "I want to be strong and healthy! And I want to join Ms. Lu's Dance Group! **I WANT TO BE A HEALTHY-DANCER KITTEN!!"** said Caldora Kitten.

"Let's go home, Mr. Frog. I have lots to tell my mom," said a happy, smiling Caldora Kitten.

When Caldora Kitten and Humphrey the Magic Frog walked to the door of her house, Caldora ran into the kitchen and called out to her mom, "Hey, Mom, you sure have one mighty smart Frog friend! Mr. Frog has given me some really good advice. And he's even gotten me to promise to drink some milk and eat some yogurt for dinner tonight."

"Why, that's wonderful, Caldora. Maybe one afternoon we can even share a snack of vanilla yogurt covered in berries," smiled Rosa Cat.

"Sure. That would be simply Purrrr-fect," said Caldora smiling her biggest, brightest smile.

Rosa Cat turned to Humphrey the Magic Frog and smiled her happiest thank-you smile.

Humphrey smiled back at Rosa Cat, tapped his nose three times, tapped his shocking-pink heart three times,

and *VANISHED* from sight!

That very night, Caldora Kitten kept her promise to Humphrey the Magic Frog. Caldora Kitten drank her very first tiny glass of milk, **"SIP, SIP, SIP, SIP."**

Caldora Kitten also ate her first tiny spoonful of yogurt. "Hmmmmmmm, good!" smiled Caldora.

Within a very short time, Caldora Kitten was drinking lots of milk and eating lots of yogurt. She now also eats other dairy products such as cottage cheese, buttermilk, soft and hard cheese, and ice cream on occasion!

Caldora Kitten also eats leafy green vegetables such as broccoli, spinach, lettuce, and kale. And she now eats salmon and sardines at least twice a week.

Caldora Kitten learned a very important lesson from her friend, Humphrey the Magic Frog. He taught her that....THERE IS MAGIC IN CALCIUM!!!

Ms. Caldora Kitten can now be found climbing the tallest trees, taking the longest steps, and Dance, Dance, Dancing with happy, kitten-like movements at Ms. Lu's School of Dance.

And as Caldora Kitten dances, twirls, bends, leaps, stretches, and bows, she can be heard humming ever-so-softly:

"MILK IS PURRRR-FECT!

MILK IS PURRRR-FECT!

MILK IS SIMPLY PURR-PURR-PURR-FECT!"

About the Author

JoAnn D. Jackovino (Ms. Jo) is an educator with over thirty years teaching experience. She has numerous teaching certifications in both New Jersey and Florida. As a teacher, Ms. Jo saw the need to help children solve their everyday problems and decided to do it in a fun, whimsical way using original animal characters to tell her stories.

A few of the topics covered in her children's stories include: Friendship, Self-Respect, Healthy Eating Habits, Proper Nutrition, Proper School Behavior, Bullying, Adoption, Family Values, and other important life-lessons for children grades Pre-K to Grade 4.

Ms. Jackovino has been writing children's stories for over twenty-five years and is presently teaching, writing, and storytelling.

You can find Ms. Jo's stories on:

CreateSpace.com
Amazon.com
magicfrogtales.com

About the Illustrator

Many thanks to artist, Hannah Fanelli, for her cover illustration. Ms. Fanelli has also illustrated *Dauntless Spirit*, a book by VSA New Jersey about Universal Design for Learning. Hannah was a co-illustrator of PLAYHOUSE VERSE, a book about original creative drama and poetry by Theatre in Motion. She has also worked as a Theatre in Motion Teaching Artist for populations with multiple disabilities. Additionally, Hannah is a professional muralist.

You can find her as a featured Teaching Artist at:

www.theatreinmotion.com

www.ingramcontent.com/pod-product-compliance
Lightning Source LLC
Chambersburg PA
CBHW041504280526
45792CB00004B/1121